Voluntarily Stopping Eating and Drinking

Voluntarily Stopping Eating and Drinking

My Wife's Ordeal

Raymond D. Smith, Jr.

Epigraph Books
Rhinebeck, New York

Cover photo by Larry Randall
Back cover photo by Gretchen Daum
Book design by Colin Rolfe

Paperback ISBN 978-1-954744-13-4
eBook ISBN 978-1-954744-14-1

Library of Congress Control Number 2021906803

Epigraph Books
22 East Market Street, Suite 304
Rhinebeck, NY 12572
(845) 876-4861
epigraphps.com

Contents

Foreword

The End

On Saturday, 7 November 2020, my wife of sixty plus years, Anne Allbright Smith, succeeded in killing herself. It took her eleven days.

At the end of 2017, she had been diagnosed with corticobasal syndrome (CBS), a somewhat rare neuro-degenerative ailment that leaves the mind relatively whole but slowly erodes the ability of muscles to function. CBS has no medications, no treatments and no cure. It is ultimately fatal.

A victim of CBS can live a long life with the disease. Someone like Anne who was otherwise in robust good health could well have lived into her hundreds. With CBS, the bulk of those years would have been in a vegetative state, confined to bed or a wheelchair, requiring others to provide all her basic needs – lifting, turning, moving, dressing, feeding, changing her diapers and cleaning her.

Anne wanted no part of such a life. Once she could no longer physically do enough of the things that made her life worth living, she determined to die.

Voluntarily stopping eating and drinking (VSED) was her only legal option.

Our pets have better deaths.

Dedication

To the early obsolescence of this volume

When Medical Aid in Dying (MAID) laws will have
been universally adopted,

When MAID's benefits will have been extended to cover
patients with terminal and fatal diseases but who may
not have a prognosis of six months or less to live

And to Anne, who went through this ordeal to achieve
her goal.

Anne Allbright Smith

Born in Chicago in 1933, Anne Allbright spent most of her comfortable upbringing in Hinsdale, Illinois, a Chicago suburb which in 1940 had a population of 7,336.

She grew up in a large house with both parents and two siblings, Joan, born in 1928 was four years seven months older and a younger brother, Bob, born in 1939. He suffered disabilities from birth and, ultimately, was sent at a very young age to live at the Devereux School in Pennsylvania which cared for and treated children and adults in similar circumstances.

With the advantage of four and a half years of seniority and – by inference, superior knowledge – Joan staked out the role of compliant, well-behaved daughter. She discovered that when she was ill, she not only was showered with attention, but also received numerous presents.

By default, Anne's place in the family was that of the often disobedient and more rebellious of the two – more adventurous and willing to try new things with alacrity. There was, for example, the time when Anne and a few friends ventured out on to the roof of her home at 632 South Elm Street in Hinsdale, IL; and the time she started a small fire when she put a towel over a table lamp to disguise the fact she was reading in bed after curfew.

As children, Joan and Anne were regularly given liver pills. Joan always appeared to take hers, while Anne protested throughout but ultimately acceded. Joan's image was modestly tarnished when a change of the dining room carpet revealed a long row of liver pills against the wall behind the sideboard. Joan had been palming and then stashing the pills.

A puppy was a longed for wish but because of beige carpeting and other concerns, was never allowed. Finally, a spaniel did join the family but was confined to the mud room and a small area of the backyard. This was not at all Anne's idea of "having a puppy."

Anne's frugality was longstanding, perhaps sparked initially by accompanying her mother on a shopping trip to Chicago. That day, her mother bought six cashmere sweaters in one go. Anne was appalled at the extravagance.

Anne spent several summers at Camp Kechua in Michigamme, MI. The camp was situated on Lake Michigamme so water sports were prominent, providing a first introduction to sailing in small boats manned by a modest crew. Music and drama, including Gilbert & Sullivan and/or take offs thereof, were also big features of camp life. Anne proudly described camp as slight on more than the essential amenities. For example, campers were housed, not in cabins but, in tents on raised platforms.

Kechua was run by three Rosses, Ella, Helen "Hy" and J. B. who at the time had some connection with Vassar College. "Hy" Ross made a deep impression on Anne as she clearly encouraged independence, self-reliance and probably nudged campers to do more than they might have thought they could.

For her final high school years, Anne was enrolled at Chatham Hall, an Episcopal girls' school in Virginia. The primary aim may have been to hone her intellectual abilities and get her into a good college. But Chatham at the time retained some of its ladies' finishing school attributes. For example, at meals, one girl oversaw each table. Her primary role was to ensure that conversation flowed evenly and that every girl was given an opportunity to speak.

The early 1950s was still a time when prep school deans or admissions advisors, had significant power over college admissions. Chatham's dean saw something in Anne and she was admitted to Vassar, when a seemingly better qualified classmate was not.

It was Anne's first time east, to a Vassar that was still all women. She was thrown into a mix of sophistication (real or posed) enhanced by the fact that many of her classmates knew each other from prep schools or social events. She had none of that built in support. Her freshman roommate, Mimi Gerstell, was from Easton, PA and flaunted it, while looking down on those from the mid-west. While majoring in English, Anne also took Russian and enjoyed tossing off Russian phrases to hall mates. Well into our marriage, I even got some of those phrases directed at me.

One college summer, Anne and a classmate got jobs as maids-of-all-work at a geology ranch in Dubois, WY. They got up pre-dawn to make breakfast; immediately thereafter made up sandwich lunches for the graduate students who would be spending the day in the field; then it was cleanup time before organizing and preparing dinner.

That stay imbued Anne with a fascination for geology. On her return to Vassar, she signed up for whatever geology courses she could fit in under the guidance of Dr. A. Scott Warthin and it became a lifetime interest. Dr. Warthin was also thesis advisor to one of Anne's classmates, Liz Cushman, whose thesis proposed what became the Student Conservation Association founded by Liz in 1957.

During her junior year at Vassar, Anne suddenly ended up overseeing Junior Party, a musical show put on by the class. She had been an assistant to the director but when the director left college, Anne inherited the job. She was initially daunted but clearly pulled it off well as was confirmed recently by a classmate. Her show was a revue entitled *Where Do We Go From Here?* and included quite a good song of the same name and a variety of skits.

Her senior year, Anne was president of the Community Religious Association, a coordinating body for the varied religious groups on campus; sponsor of a weekend religious conference; and a facilitator for volunteer work in Poughkeepsie's welfare centers.

It was for one such conference that Anne was hostess to Paul Tillich, professor of theology at New York City's Union Theological Seminary. She would have mentioned to Dr, Tillich that she had applied to Union for admission but had not yet had a response. Soon after Dr. Tillich's return to the city, Anne got a letter of acceptance.

Finally, as she later put it, "BOYS!" Well, yes, but this was also a time when Union's faculty included such greats as Dr. Tillich, Paul Meilenburg and others. She also enjoyed the whole New York City scene. In 1958, Anne graduated from Union with a B.D., later upgraded to an M.Div. But, what to do? She was an Episcopalian at a time when that church did not ordain women.

She took a job as a teacher's assistant at the Day School of the Church of the Heavenly Rest at Fifth Avenue and 90th Street in New York and shared a fifth floor walkup apartment on 88th Street between Park and Lexington Avenues with a Union classmate, Lucy Ward.

Anne's application for a Bloomingdale's charge account asked for her annual salary which she listed as $2,000. The application was declined. I suggested that she resubmit her application but leave the salary question unanswered. Her application was promptly approved.

I met Anne soon after I got out of the Army in September 1958, just as she was starting her job at the Day School. By the end of 1958, I had a $95 a week job as a trainee at Bankers Trust Company in the city. As another English major, I was fortunate that BTCo had a two year training program. With that, night courses at NYU and a bit of diligence, I was transformed into a commercial banker.

Anne and I were married in August 1960 at the Church of the Heavenly Rest. We had managed to find a rent controlled two bedroom eighth floor corner apartment at 93rd Street and Lexington Avenue. The rent was $160.43 per month. There were a few drawbacks: Lexington Avenue was still two way, so there were nightly episodes of fire engines racing up and down the avenue, punctuated especially on weekends by raucous patrons of the Irish bar across the street. Over time, we were able to tune all that out.

We were dissimilar in small ways but not the important ones. Anne was impetuous and quick to make decisions. I was inclined to ponder a decision from many angles, even a word in a simple note. When Anne put a pot on to cook it was always set to high. She would adjust later. I would put the pot on medium and make sure nothing might burn. Anne's method was quicker; mine slower but with less chance things would boil over.

We wanted children but when none were forthcoming, we adopted Randy as an infant in the spring of 1966.

I had to move my "office," which had occupied our second bedroom, into a corner of our apartment. Having grown up in the suburbs I wanted out of the city in due course, but we had many friends there and Anne was less inclined to leave. What did it for her was returning from Central Park one day with Randy in his carriage. The white blanket with which he was covered was liberally peppered with soot.

In April 1967, we moved to a home in Pound Ridge, NY about twelve miles due north of Stamford, CT from which (among other places) I could get a train into the city. The round trip commute consumed three hours of each workday. But now, with a home of our own, dogs soon entered the family. They were given complete run of the house and environs and have been part of our family ever since.

Anne had become pregnant and in October 1967, gave birth to Becca at Stamford Hospital, which was the only nearby hospital at the time that both favored the Lamaze method of childbirth and admitted a spouse into the delivery room. We both insisted on the latter and Anne had to change both her obstetrician and our original hospital to achieve those goals. As she grew, Becca tired of my occasional taunt, "Listen, kid, the first time I saw you, you were greenish gray and slimy."

The summer of 1968 found Anne, Randy and Becca at the Pound Ridge Town Park where they first met Ginny Powers and her two children, Jonathan and David. They were almost the same ages as our two. Ginny and Jon Powers became and have remained lifelong friends.

Early on, Randy's interest in becoming a drummer manifested itself when he formed an impromptu band with friends banging on boxes, garbage can lids and playing a few horns. He acquired a drum set and took a few lessons from our next door neighbor, Brian Smith. As his interest in rock music and composing grew, Randy shifted more to the guitar, acoustic and electric and acquired more sound equipment.

By age eight, Becca had learned the conventions of letter writing. What my transgression was, neither of us can now remember, but I was handed a short note reading: "Dear Daddy I hate you love, Rebecca."

Anne became a member of the Pound Ridge Recreation Commission, chaired by her friend, Tally Nordheim. She was thus able to help shape several innovative town programs for children.

When Randy and Becca grew older, we began taking summer trips out west to visit our national parks. The dogs couldn't come, but another important member of the family from whom Becca was inseparable could. Gray Bear had been acquired probably when she was a toddler, perhaps even as a crib toy. Over the years his fur and his name had been worn down so he was now plain Graybe.

On one western trip, Zion National Park was our last stop before heading to Las Vegas for a flight home. We left Zion and had driven maybe twenty or thirty minutes when we discovered Graybe was not with us. There was no need for pleading by Becca. As one, we agreed and I simply turned the car around and sped back to Zion. We knew where Graybe had last been with us and quickly discovered him perched in a gnarled tree. Back we sped toward Vegas. I was stopped for speeding and we probably missed our flight but we had recovered the treasured bear.

Ever after, when anyone in the family was missing something, one or another of us would almost always opine, "Lost in a tree at Zion."

As Randy and Becca progressed in school, it became obvious that a traditional school environment was not ideal for Randy. To have a say in the outcome, Anne became a member of our school district's Committee on the Handicapped. This Committee encouraged Anne to explore options for Randy and in due course she hit upon the Rhinebeck Country School which Randy attended from June 1979 until June 1981.

In 1982 to celebrate Randy's sixteenth birthday, he and I took an ambitious two week July trip through France. The impetus was to celebrate the occasion, of course, but also to give Randy a trip overseas to a country I loved. At its end, my contemporary summation of the trip reads: ". . . too much total driving, 4,529 kilometers or 2,808 miles – the weather has been fine though a bit hot at the beginning. We've seen a lot of great stuff, but best of all, we've gotten better acquainted and learned a bit about each other and our differing points of view on a lot of subjects but similar on a lot of others (both negative on guided tours)." Randy had been dismayed there were no delis in France. Did he really need a grinder? On the other hand, he was delighted he could be served beer with no questions asked.

Randy returned to his mainstream high school at which Becca was excelling but where he continued to have frustrations. Though Anne and I came from education-centric families, both we and Randy soon agreed this was not working out and that his desire to drop out of high school and move to Hadley, MA to share an apartment with a contemporary, made a certain amount of sense.

Becca had become increasingly interested in horses and horseback riding at Echo Farm in South Salem, NY which was owned by Al Ridgeway, a veteran of World War II, who was assisted by Madelyn Kuntz. Al presided and did the maintenance of fields, barns and fences, but left the horse care and teaching to Madelyn, who taught Becca to ride.

A routine was established: when Becca returned from school, it was off to Echo Farm for the afternoon where she rode and tended the horse she rode. This led her into the Goldens Bridge Hounds Pony Club (GBHPC) for which Anne eventually became US Pony Clubs (USPC) District Commissioner. This pony club was attached to the Goldens Bridge Hounds hunt.

One early winter day, Becca joined a GBH fox hunt, meeting that day at the home of William Randolph Hearst

III. It was still dark as the hunt assembled on the spacious front lawn with the white columns of the main house just visible on a slight rise. Snow had started to fall and Irish coffee with real whipped cream was being served to riders and observers alike. For a few moments, one could forget the excess, imagine being back at an English country house a century earlier and just enjoy the scene and the riders in jackets of scarlet and black against the white of the snowfall.

Anne thought it would be better to have a pony club centered at Echo Farm. So, she figured out how to do that and founded Honey Hollow Pony Club (HHPC) for that purpose and ultimately became USPC's Metro Region supervisor.

As she watched Becca ride off on one hunter pace, Anne vowed she would not be left out again. She took riding lessons and was on that same pace a year later. When Becca went to college in the fall of 1985, Anne inherited Becca's pony, Wishful Thinkin'.

In the summer of 1986, just months before the bank transferred me to its London office, we bought a Pound Ridge home on a bit less than five acres. The attraction was that it had both a small barn and a modest riding ring. Wish could thus be kept at home with us, saving boarding fees. A drawback, of course, was that Anne became stall mucker-out-in-chief.

Not surprisingly, when we went to London, Anne insisted that not only our dog, Brownie, but Wishful

Thinkin' had to come too. As it happened, Wish arrived at her new farm home before we arrived in England. The barn manager told us, "I've been trying to talk American to Wish to get her more easily accustomed to us."

Bringing the pony was a fortuitous decision as the pony immediately gave Anne entrée into English life via South Medburn Farm, where she was stabled. At the farm, where she rode nearly every day, Anne made another life-long friend, Jean Cass. Together, they would ride out for lunch at a nearby pub or just wander trails on the 105 acre farm.

We returned to our Pound Ridge home in 1989, the year Becca graduated from college. Becca had been bereft of a dog in college so almost immediately adopted Sid, a stray about eight months old found wandering the streets of Somers, NY. Becca soon had a job at Guadalupe National Park in Texas; but, she would not be able to take Sid, so he joined Brownie as our second dog.

Anne noticed that Sid often jumped the horse jumps in the ring just for fun. We had seen demonstrations of dog agility while in England and thought that would be a good way to channel Sid's energy. She learned more; found no agility clubs nearby, but did find Laurie Ward, just across the line in Ridgefield, CT, who knew something about dog agility and convinced her that the two of them should start Contact Agility Club. Sid earned a wall full of ribbons crowned by being a finalist in the U. S. Dog Agility Association Nationals in 1996. Anne wrote, "Along the way, he taught me a thing or two about patience, caring and persistence."

About this time Anne had discovered the fascination of birding. With typical determination, she set out to identify all the local birds by sight and then to perfect her skills at identifying them solely by the sounds of their calls. With our friends the Powers, we made several birding trips to Central and South America, for each of which Anne prepared carefully, studying types and markings of birds we were likely to encounter and their sounds, as well.

At some point, we had acquired a mixed breed rescue dog who was largely Australian cattle dog (ACD). This high drive breed fascinated Anne and she enjoyed working with our new pet named Dingo. Unfortunately, we soon discovered that at any opportunity, Dingo would attack Sid which meant we had to keep them apart. Not always an easy job. Dingo also developed several maladies which we treated but, ultimately, he had to be put down. Anne vowed to replace him with a pure bred ACD she could acquire close to birth and train herself.

Not long after I retired in 1992, we began hiking in the Shawangunk Mountains near Gardiner, NY, seventy miles northwest of Pound Ridge. The dogs loved it and we went usually once a week and often twice. One day while jogging, I thought, why don't we move to Gardiner and save the trip. Anne agreed. Our friends were surprised, especially after so many years in Pound Ridge. But Pound Ridge was changing, too.

We think we found the last best vacant land in Gardiner when we bought 62.4 acres in 2002. We then retained Gardiner architect Matthew Bialecki to design a cypress, stone and glass home which afforded us a panoramic view of the sheer rock face of the Shawangunk Mountains four miles distant. The design process was a test of our marriage as Anne was happy to entertain some of Matt's extreme fantasies that could take me weeks to back out of the design drawings, once Anne (finally) and I agreed they were too over the top and clearly too expensive. David Kucera, also of Gardiner, contracted to build the house and in April, 2004, we moved into our still incomplete new home.

During construction, an eastern box turtle was discovered near the house. More turned up and Anne became increasingly fascinated with these creatures and started recording her findings.

In the fall of 2003, she had acquired eight week old Anzac, a pure bred Australian cattle dog (ACD). Unlike Australian shepherds, ACDs were actually bred in Australia to herd cattle and include in their lineage the dingo. Depending on coloring they are also referred to as blue or red heelers as their herding technique is to nip at the heels of the cattle they are controlling. They are smart, tough, intelligent and trainable working dogs. But you need to train or otherwise work with them all the time or they will find their own ways to expend energy. These may not coincide with yours.

The Hudson Valley Tracking Club was based nearby

and here was a whole new dog sport. Unlike most, where the handler directs what the dog does, in tracking only the dog knows what to do. By simply walking a tracking course, an individual lays down a scent. The dog is brought to the starting line, offered something to smell that was recently handled by the track layer, like an old sock, to pick up the proper scent and then sent off on the course with the handler at the other end of a long lead line. Anzac became an excellent, deliberate and methodical tracking dog and was joined four years later by another eight week old ACD pup, Diggy.

Diggy became a good tracking dog, as well, but was much more impetuous, occasionally missing a turn in a track because she was going too fast, or just following a track and then suddenly veering off to run around in a tight circle out of sheer exuberance before returning to the work at hand.

As Anzac and Diggy matured and their personalities became clearer, I gave them nicknames suitable to those distinct personalities. Anzac was first Anzac Smith or Dog Smith, in keeping with his more formal dignity. In old age, he became Big Fuzzy, like a big teddy bear. Literally and figuratively, Diggy was harder to pin down, becoming variously The Wig because she wiggled so much or DigBat because that's what she was. Diggy, who mirrored some of Anne's traits, became my "special dog" and Anzac, whose demeanor was closer to mine, became Anne's "best buddy."

It didn't take long for Anne to realize she could enlist Anzac and Diggy to help her track the eastern box turtles on our property when the vegetation was high and the ground not easily viewed by humans. The dogs got the hang of it quickly and became invaluable. This teamwork Anne documented in her book, *The Silence of the Bell: Monitoring Eastern Box Turtles with Australian Cattle Dogs* (2015), available on Amazon.

We had already been hiking for some time with our dogs but then we discovered geocaching. You use GPS coordinates and a limited number of clues to find hidden items, often in parks or similar areas. The caches drew us to wonderful spots we might not otherwise have found and once within ten yards or so of the cache location, based on the coordinates, Anzac and Diggy would often be the first to find the actual cache. These forays nearly always included Ginny and Jon Powers and a morning of geocaching was always followed by a good lunch at a carefully selected restaurant.

With a new home in Gardiner, again, we figured we would always stay there. We were aware of Woodland Pond, a continuing care retirement community (CCRC) just eight miles away. Anne's sister, Joan and husband Jim Ashley, lived at one in New Hampshire. We vowed never to live at a place like that.

Later, we thought, when one of us died, the other would not want to continue living back in the woods on a dead end road with a driveway a third of a mile long. We gave Woodland Pond a closer look and in March, 2011 we paid an entrance fee for Cottage 8 and became residents. Increasingly, our activities shifted to Woodland Pond – watching beavers at their beaver pond, swimming laps in the indoor pool, serving on their Mill Brook Preserve Committee, meals with friends in the dining room, etc. Some days we made three trips over and back home for various events. Anne became a member and secretary of the Residents' Council and I was one of the first two residents selected for the newly independent Woodland Pond board of directors in June 2016.

A motion sensitive camera enabled us to film animals at the beaver pond 24/7. These short takes Anne spliced into what became four annual video presentations, "What's Happening at the Beaver Pond," which delighted residents and elicited thoughtful questions. She also started keeping track of various turtles found on the Woodland Pond campus.

Diagnosis of Corticobasal Syndrome (CBS)

By 2017, both Anne and I were experiencing moderate balance issues. We had been seeing Dr. Ravichandra Reddy, a physical medicine and rehabilitation specialist. Anne was having more mobility and balance difficulties and Ravi recommended that she see a therapist at MidHudson Regional Hospital's Therapy Connection. Anne worked with him for several months and it was he who may first have sensed the possibility that she might suffer from a neuro-degenerative ailment of some sort.

In late June that summer, Anne fell backward while stepping up from our patio into the house, cutting a deep gash in her head. A visit to the emergency room required six staples to close the wound and indicated she might have fractured two ribs. There was, however, no evidence of concussion. The incident increased our concerns about balance.

Anne was also having increasing difficulty walking and, though I could not detect it in her spoken words, she said she was finding it more and more difficult quickly to find, frame and then speak the words she wanted to say. This frustration was compounded whenever others started finishing her sentences.

Neither of us had ever consulted a neurologist and to get a better fix on Anne's condition, Ravi recommended that Anne see a well-regarded Poughkeepsie neurologist. A New York City friend who was herself a noted neurologist knew and confirmed that the recommended neurologist was a skilled diagnostician.

Anne saw him at least twice in December 2017. After the second appointment on 22 December, he wanted to confirm his findings with colleagues (including our friend). He was leaving shortly on a skiing vacation in Canada but assured us that he was reachable and would let us know his conclusions as soon as he had confirmed them.

We heard nothing though we learned later that "someone had tried to call us" on 22 December. On 27 December we phoned the doctor's office and a member of his staff, informed us the diagnosis was corticobasal syndrome (CBS). We had never heard of it. The doctor was still away but this news launched us into our own research on the nature and prognosis for CBS before our next appointment with him on 19 January 2018.

On 19 January, the doctor told us he had suspected CBS, which he described as a "Parkinsonism that doesn't respond well to medicine." He had made a few short film clips of Anne walking and shared them and his notes with colleagues at Mt. Sinai, including with our own neurologist friend and summed up the collective wisdom, "If Ruth thought it and I thought it was corticobasal syndrome, it's pretty definitive."

There is no medical treatment and no medicine to treat or slow CBS. The only things the doctor could offer were scrips for occupational therapy for hands and legs. He also suggested Anne might be accepted into a study for a slightly related ailment, but that would require trips into Manhattan. NFW.

After fifteen or twenty minutes in his office, the ever-practical doctor became dismissive. He had diagnosed the ailment; he could do nothing useful for it; so there seemed little reason for us to hang around. We left.

Ataxia, the presence of abnormal, uncoordinated movements, had already been part of the neurologist's diagnosis but at this appointment he also used the term apraxia, the inability to perform some purposive actions because of brain damage. Could this be the result of Anne's fall in June 2017 and/or the pernicious stealth of CBS?

Sunday, 30 September 2018 was not a good day for Anne. At one point she was having a lot of trouble balancing, working her fingers properly; and some difficulty walking. She found that it was all getting too difficult and finally her face just crumpled up near to tears and she said, "I can't go on like this – period." I helped her to a seat. She sat down and began to recover somewhat. But these things happened more and more frequently. Around this time, Anne said she thought she might have been exhibiting signs of CBS as long ago as 2015 when we went to my college reunion and she suddenly could not use the escalators at Dulles International Airport.

The end of December 2018, Anne and I were walking down our driveway when she fell, put out her arm to break her fall and broke her left wrist. Although Anne wrote with her left hand, she could do most things equally well with her right and was able to make do while wearing a cast and later a brace. With her left hand temporarily out of commission and her right arm and several fingers of her right hand already impacted by CBS, Anne now needed a wheelchair. We borrowed one from Woodland Pond until 9 January 2019 when Anne's Pride Mobility Go Go Elite Traveler power scooter was delivered to the house.

We had not planned to move to our cottage at Woodland Pond until both dogs died. But Anne's increasing incapacities and the dogs' good health made us change our plans. In January 2019, we began discussing with Patrick Sheehan of Sotheby's selling our home.

In a flurry of action and with the invaluable assistance of Colleen Ashe of Ashe Organizing Solutions, we managed to get the house cleaned up; dumpster loads of trash cleared out; and salvageable items donated to charity. We moved to our cottage in May 2019 and put the house on the market in early summer. It sold within a week to a Brooklyn couple who were perfectly happy with a conservation easement on the property and have since become good friends.

We developed new routines at Woodland Pond where we already knew many residents. The dogs seemed to adjust fine to their new surroundings and we could easily take them on walks down the gravel track next to our cottage. This relative calm was shattered that summer when Diggy was diagnosed with lymphoma and given a prognosis of mere days to live. Though she remained energetic till the last, her swollen lymph glands made it increasingly difficult for her to breathe. This may have caused the hacking sneezing/cough, especially prevalent at night. We put her down Saturday morning, 26 October 2019.

That afternoon, Anne wrote to concerned friends, "Sad news. Last night Diggy had trouble breathing all night long which meant that nobody got any sleep at all . . . she would breathe ever so heavily and then get up and walk around coughing and panting like there was no tomorrow. There was no question about what to do.

"Our vet Eric is away at a dog show but I don't think that Diggy cared at all when a different vet appeared because she was much too busy begging for chicken snaps from me, her bright little face as animated and excited as usual. She didn't even notice the sedative going into her leg and then she was too sedated to care about the second shot. No nervousness or anxiety, simple and fast.

"But it breaks my heart watching Anzac going around and around the cottage looking for her. We did stop at the house on the way home to let him sniff around and he seemed pleased with this and we were pleased to see Robert and Jill, who had invited us over this morning.

"I can't believe that just five weeks ago we thought Diggy was going to live forever. How fast lymphoma sneaks in and spreads. It will be some time before I can believe that she is really gone. I just hope Anzac doesn't go in the meantime.

"What a great little dog she was – so lively, so eager to do anything. I feel as though somebody took my head and stomped on it."

Years before, we had made plans for Diggy to live with our daughter in full expectation that she would outlive us both. Her sudden death was a huge blow to all three of us, including Anzac, who wandered the cottage for days trying to find Diggy. Some months later Anne announced after an especially stressful day that she would stick around until Anzac died but that after that, she would voluntarily stop eating and drinking (VSED).

From our weekly visits to the Health Center, Anne had noticed several residents with mobility problems and thought an occasional meeting to discuss together coping techniques might benefit all. Within days and the help of the Health Center 's Activities Director, Marin Lott, she had such a group meeting monthly.

Anne's ability to walk declined steadily and a better power chair was needed, since she was now largely 'confined to bed or her chair. In April 2020, she acquired a Quickee Q500M power wheelchair with a list price above the cost of any car we had ever owned. This could tilt and recline, making it much more comfortable for a full day's use. The dining table was swapped for one that would allow the new chair to get closer. Anne's desk was raised so the chair could better approach her keyboard. Efforts were made to find utensils that would make feeding herself easier.

The end of April, a hospital bed was shoehorned into the bedroom next to our queen sized bed. Because of its adjustability, Anne was better able to control her sleeping positions as she could no longer turn on her own. Even so, she was never able to get truly comfortable and fell into no better than fitful sleep.

In early May 2020, Kim Sylvester started coming twice a week to wash Anne's hair and Ana Flores became a mainstay each weekday, helping us between 7 and 9AM and again between 5 and 8PM at night. Their dependability and help were invaluable but even more uplifting were the smiles and cheerful outlook each brought to our cottage.

Anzac, who would be seventeen in September 2020 was more visibly slowing down.

He was less and less interested in the short walks our dog walker took him on twice a day. As summer began, his interest in food declined. He slept most of the time and ate little. Thankfully, his long-time vet, Eric Hartelius, DVM, was able to come to the cottage to put him down on Wednesday, 1 July 2020. Anzac, who had been with us since the age of eight weeks was our last dog and Anne's last living link with the dog activities that had been her life. His loss clearly accelerated her decline. Pictures of both Anzac and Diggy throughout the cottage were constant reminders of their absence.

We both knew this was coming. We had plenty of warning. But it was a final blow to Anne . . . her last living link with the vital, outdoor dog oriented life she had led for so many years. Her "best buddy" was now gone.

Anne wrote: "Our vet came to our cottage yesterday to put Anzac down. He would have been seventeen years old in September. He was not in pain, but he wanted to sleep all day long, not go outside, and not eat. So, we all agreed it was time to say goodbye.

"I learned most of what I know about dog behavior from him. He was very special, and that is an understatement. He leaves an enormous hole in our hearts and lives."

Anne had continued movement therapy with the addition of speech therapy and individual practice using the Parkinson Voice Project. The latter particularly appealed as Anne was a member of Woodland Pond's choral group, the Pondaliers, and the Parkinson Voice Project fostered choruses of voice impaired individuals worldwide.

These therapies were helpful in coping with CBS but none did anything to recover lost skills. Sometimes, I thought they only served as a means of "doing something" even as we knew nothing would stop, slow or reverse the progression of CBS.

As the weeks passed, a routine was established with Ana. Because of space limitations, it had something of the ballet about it, the three of us each playing our part. On arrival at 7AM, Ana would strip off Anne's urine soaked Assurance; I would be close at hand with a *New York Times* home delivery plastic bag into which Ana would neatly slide the Assurance which I would then tie and dump in the garbage. While Ana was sponge bathing Anne's perineum, I would navigate her power chair into the bedroom alongside the bed. To the extent possible, Ana would dress Anne while she was still in bed. Despite her short stature, Ana was extraordinarily strong and once Anne was helped to stand and dressing completed, Ana was able to lift and turn Anne enough to sit in her power chair. Ana would then organize breakfast for us and clean up.

Before Ana left at 9AM Anne would try to use the commode in the kitchen as that was the most open area and would accommodate the commode, power chair and at least the two people now required to help Anne use it safely. Occasionally, we weren't quick enough and that would require cleanup of varying degrees of complexity. Going from a life of constant activity to being nearly totally sedentary required careful management to avoid constipation. Too much Duralax could create sudden diarrhea. Getting to the commode instantly was no longer possible.

We both enjoyed meals with friends in the dining room especially at lunch, but these now had to be carefully orchestrated. In good weather it was easy for Anne to ride to the dining room in her power chair; lift the arms of the chair so that it could drive in close to the table; put on her bib and have a limited meal.

A week before Anne started to VSED we had just such a lunch in the dining room with another couple. Because of her increasing limitations, the meal had to be a thin sandwich Anne could easily hold with one hand. A grilled cheese was really the only option as the contents of the sandwich would not slide out the other side when you took a first bite. A drink with a straw was doable but it was all increasingly frustrating to Anne.

Confinement to bed or a power chair, especially as the weather cooled and more time was spent inside in warmer, dryer air, took its toll on Anne's skin. Itching was treated with Gold Bond Body Powder. Against dry skin, we marshalled lip balm, lanolin rich Bag Balm, Curél lotion and Balmex cream. It was a never-ending effort to keep her skin lubricated and itch free. There were Tylenol and Aleve for a persistent pain in the back of Anne's head when in bed. And there were Robitussin and cough drops for an occasional cough that could keep her awake. A Vicks humidifier helped diminish the dry air in the bedroom.

The simple operation of going to bed could occupy much of an hour, especially trying to get Anne's head comfortable against her pillow. Different pillows were tried. There was also a tendency for her head to loll left and this was dealt with by stuffing old rags (cloth diapers that had survived many moves, dishtowels, etc.) beside her head. Once more or less settled, bedtime ended with my reading a few pages from A. A. Milne's *The House at Pooh Corner*, an often funny, sometimes sly depiction of human nature that's never lost its relevance. In old age, as it was when we were very small, the book has a wonderful time-for-bed soothing tone.

I was amused recently to read in John Tusa's book about boardroom management, *On Board* (2020), a description of a particularly weak board as one made up largely of "Rabbit and all his friends and relations."

Sometime around mid-October, while Dr. Maggie Carpenter was visiting via Skype, Anne announced, "I'm going to start VSED." Maggie's response was, "You're a very brave woman." I didn't understand that response then. I do now.

Anne's VSED Ordeal

Anne's sister Joan had caused her own death in 2015 by VSED. She was in skilled nursing at Kendal in Hanover, NH and made an extended party out of the event, inviting friends and relations to visit before she started. We drove up to see her one last time. She gathered all her children to her, ensuring that at least one sat with her throughout, available to rub ice on her lips. She was in pain so the morphine dose got upped frequently. It took her eleven days to die.

The one book we had found on the subject was *Choosing to Die: A Personal Story, Elective Death by Voluntarily Stopping Eating and Drinking (VSED) in the Face of Degenerative Disease* by Phyllis Shacter. This painted a rosy picture of the process and we were busy so did not inquire further or do a lot more research.

Anne could still get around and get into the car and we were still able to have meals with friends, go places and do other things important to us. Nonetheless it was apparent that CBS was continuing to take its toll.

Early in 2019, we began to make plans to move to our cottage at Woodland Pond in New Paltz (NY). We managed to clean up the house; move in May of that year; put the house on the market that summer; and sell it within a week.

In September 2019, at a vet appointment it was discovered that Diggy had lymphoma. This was an unexpected blow to both of us. Diggy was just twelve years old and we had long assumed Diggy might outlive both of us.

Despite remaining frisky up till the end, Diggy was having trouble breathing and we put her down in October of 2019. This was hard to recover from. On a gray fall day, we scattered her ashes on the agility field at our old house where she had been a star.

The right side of Anne's body exhibited the most symptoms of CBS – her right foot was less maneuverable; the fingers on her right hand lost responsiveness; and her right arm slowly became rigid against her body. Chores requiring two hands became impossible without help.

The kitchen had always been Anne's domain, though I helped with particular specialties of my own, like grilling flank steak. We ate some dinners in the Woodland Pond dining room but for the most part, preferred Anne's cooking. She had been quick, efficient and invariably produced tasty meals though some "experiments" panned out better than others. Now, she could do nothing but watch, direct or suggest as I tried to prepare or more often simply organize our dinners.

One evening with the intent of steaming some peas, I pulled out the double boiler I used for that purpose. Anne said, "You have to use the bigger one with the two handles." I declined, explaining the smaller had a glass top lid so I could see at a glance how things were going and we weren't steaming a lot of peas.

Anne's fury at that point was out of all proportion. I could only gape, until I realized it was not directed at me (as she later confirmed). It was directed at a disease that had left her skills of a lifetime "unusable."

She recovered her composure. But how, and why? She was not going to get better. Her future was nearing its bleakest.

Even reading a book, a simple pastime we all take for granted, became more difficult for Anne. Think a minute about the mechanics. You hold a book in one or two hands but when it comes time to turn a page, one hand holds the book while the other flips the page. How can you easily do that if one hand doesn't really function? To simplify this for Anne, we acquired over time various options – hand weights to hold down the pages; a book stand; and stands for the book with arms that came out to hold the pages flat. But every time a page needed turning, you still needed two hands.

Audio books became a more workable solution. But your freedom was still restricted as they did not always offer the titles Anne was interested in. A further shrinkage in the range of Anne's life.

For much of one's life, we count on things "improving." We'll finally build our dream house. If I just train better I'll be able to run a 10K in under forty minutes. When I take this pill, my ailment will be cured. By the time we are surprised to find ourselves correctly classed as "elderly," all of that is gone. We're not expecting to get dramatically better. We're just hoping to hang on to what we have or slow various declines like weakening eyesight, poorer hearing, loss of strength, stamina and balance. Life becomes one of modest goals with few classed as achievements.

Suppose that, superimposed on the above, you had an untreatable, incurable, steadily progressing disorder that would ultimately kill you. But not before leaving you in a state where your mind was fine but physically, you could do next to nothing without the assistance of others. Loss of independence is among the most devastating to the elderly.

Early in 2020, protection against the covid-19 virus became all consuming, especially in New York state where the virus had spiked. By March, Woodland Pond was in some form of lockdown with meals, mail and other necessities brought directly to our cottage. We were still able to get out and drive a bit, though it was increasingly difficult for Anne to get into and out of the car because of balance issues.

Anne was having more and more difficulty with her voice -- framing her words properly and, when dictating, generating the correct words on her computer monitor.

With meals cut into bite size pieces, she could still feed herself. Most activities of daily life required some assistance from me, which I had so far been able to provide.

By early summer, we had signed up Ana Flores and Kim Sylvester to help take care of Anne during the day. Kim came for an hour each Monday and Friday morning to wash Anne's hair and Ana came from 7 until 9 in the morning and from 5 until 8 in the evening during the week and greatly simplified our lives.

Anzac, who would be seventeen in September, was becoming more sluggish and, sleeping more. Finally, it was obvious to both of us that it was time for him to go and we put him down on 1 July 2020. Fortunately, his longtime vet was able to come to the cottage so there was no need to move Anzac from familiar surroundings.

In a year of tragedies, Anzac's death was the worst. For Anne, he was her "best buddy" – the last living link with the outdoor, dog-centric life that she normally led. Even when she went on brief errands, the dogs always had to be loaded into the car to go along. Now there were no more dogs to load. It left Anne with a further sense of her life shrinking.

Anne asked me when she should start VSED and I told her that was a decision that had to be entirely her own , even though I and our children all supported her plans. We obviously wanted her to stay with us as long as she thought her life had meaning.

In October of 2020, Anne announced that she was

going to start VSED. Her doctor told her, "You're a very brave woman." I was surprised by that comment at the time. I understand it now.

Dinner in our cottage on Tuesday evening, 27 October was Anne's last food and drink. I have no recollection of the meal but it did include wine.

VSED Diary and Medications

Care Givers:
    Weekdays
        Ana Flores: 7AM – 9AM and 5PM – 8PM
        Sonia Flores: 9PM – 6AM
    Weekends
        Gwen Wright: 7AM – 8PM

Medications Used:
    Aleve (Naproxen sodium) 220 mg each
    Ativan (Lorazepam)
    Gin
    Haldol
    Medical Marijuana
    Morphine
    Oxycodone
    Quetiapine
    Tylenol (Acetaminophen) 500mg each

Day One: Wednesday, 28 Oct 20

12:00AM – 1 Ativan + 1 marijuana.

I had an early morning ophthalmologist appointment in Kingston, NY. Anne had no problems not eating or drinking. She did not normally drink that much anyway but was surprised at the lack of hunger pangs. She didn't even mind watching me eat. The day passed more or less normally.

6:30PM – 1 Ativan

Day Two: Thursday, 29 Oct 20

Sarah Tolchin, Hospice RN, who would be our case manager visited in the late morning.

She suggested wet sponges on sticks to moisten the membranes of Anne's mouth.

Soon after, we hit upon the spray bottle used on our orchids as a better option.

Hospice oxygen and other equipment arrived in the late afternoon.

Day Three: Friday, 30 Oct 20

Kim Sylvester came in the morning and washed Anne's hair.

6:35PM When we phoned seeking options, hospice nurse Richard said we could rinse Anne's mouth often with Biotene to keep it moist.

Day Four: Saturday, 31 Oct 20

We had a hard frost overnight with the temperature in the twenties in the morning.

Nonetheless, we went for a power chair ride wearing gloves.

Day Five: Sunday, 1 Nov 20

Anne had a bad night and her voice was faint in the morning.

The morning was cold but above freezing.

When the temperature got into high 40s, even though there was a light, gray rain, Anne wanted to go out in the power chairs. So we put on rain gear, plastic bags over the chair controls and set out. We didn't last too long.

Late afternoon, Becca returned from Colorado.

We watched "Sound of Music" that evening.

Day Six: Monday, 2 Nov 20

Fitful sleep for Anne last night.

The day was sunny, blustery, windy and cold.

Sarah Tolchin came by mid-afternoon in her space suit.

Maggie Carpenter came by 4:30PM; "Gin?" ... "Why not?"; Morphine as needed.

Can take 1 Ativan, 1 morphine + 1 marijuana every 4 hours; if more is needed, can up the dosages to 2 every 4 hours.

Can give more liquid marijuana than just the bulb of the syringe; when it runs out, don't bother renewing.

Day Seven: Tuesday, 3 Nov 20

10:15AM Sarah Tolchin came by and concurred with the above upped doses.

She suggested giving doses regularly every 4 hours rather than just on demand.

11:30AM Maggie called: every 4 hours 2 Ativan, 0.5mL morphine and marijuana if asked for or needed until it runs out. Also, spray water inside Anne's mouth but wait thirty minutes after giving medications. Once Anne's asleep, stop the medications.

12:49PM Anne was resting quietly.

We hoped to get Anne to sleep more which she did off and on during the day.

She made lots of demands but we hoped the new regime would work.

She never said so but maybe she was hanging on to get the election results.

We got Anne to bed about 6ish but she was never comfortable and never really slept.

Day Eight: Wednesday, 4 Nov 20

From 1:18 – 3:35AM we were all up with Anne's demands for water and wanting to get out of bed and sit in her power chair.

Finally she slept slumped over until about 6:30AM.

The election seemed hung up at 227 to 213 electoral votes of the 270 needed to win.

Sarah Tolchin came by about 10AM.

She and Maggie prescribed 0.50mL Haldol + 1.0mL morphine every 4 hours and it did have a calming effect.

Anne was now too weak to swallow water with pills.

Liquid Lorazepam (Ativan) arrived at 3:30PM.

Anne had diarrhea in her pants before we could get her onto the commode.

Ana arrived, cleaned up Anne, settled her and by 6:50PM she was sleeping soundly.

Becca made short work of Childe Hassam's complex "Flags on 57th Street" jigsaw puzzle.

Day Nine: Thursday, 5 Nov 20

Sarah Tolchin came by about 10AM.

At 1:55PM, Anne awoke.

At 2:00PM, we gave her medicine.

At 2:05PM, while coughing, she asked, "Can I sit up?"

At 2:15PM, her eyes opened and she said to me, "Don't go away."

By 3:00PM, she was restless but less so than an hour before.

Day Ten: Friday, 6 Nov 20

Anne was in a coma and unresponsive.
Sarah Tolchin came by about 10AM.
Maggie Carpenter came by about 1PM.

Day Eleven: Saturday, 7 Nov 20

11:50AM I told Anne that Biden had won. She gave no sign of hearing.

1:50 PM, Anne stopped breathing and died while Becca and I were having lunch.

Gina Law, RN, Hospice nurse on duty came. She put these details in the medical record:

> **Date/time of death:** Nov 7, 2020 14:42:00
> **Location:** Pt's home with spouse and daughter at bedside
> **Notifications:** Coroner Notified; Verified Bereaved Information; Visit made; Notified attending physician; Notified medical director; Prepared body prior to removal; Notified mortuary; Disposed of medications; Protocol followed for medication disposal; Initiated equipment pick-up; Assisted family with mortuary pick-up.

Anne had been in a coma. The skin, tight across her skull, was a waxy yellow gray; her eyes mere slits; and her mouth gaped open revealing the dehydrated blackness within. I was reminded of a beached fish in its final moments. There was no sense of a peaceful or painless death.

The absence of food was not the blunt instrument of VSED; in fact it seemed of little consequence to Anne. The lack of fluid intake led to her death as that deprivation degraded and then shut down bodily functions.

Our bodies are about 60% water and during a day, we're liable to lose via breath, sweat, urine, feces, tears, spit or nose blowing as much as three quarts of water. If that's not regularly replaced, your body rations what water it retains. Your urine becomes darker because kidneys send less diluting water to your bladder; blood gets thicker and slower; and your heart must pump harder to maintain oxygen levels.

Maintaining blood pressure gets more and more difficult. To compensate, the body slows blood flow to less vital organs, like the kidneys and intestines, damaging these organs as waste builds up.

We tried to mitigate Anne's pain and discomfort with drugs and by moistening her mouth. But the pain and discomfort were never more than marginally reduced. During the eleven day VSED process, Anne was never ever comfortable or pain free.

Monday, 9 November at 5:15AM Becca left for Albany Airport to return home.

Tuesday, 10 November at 4:30PM, Jim Sullivan, one of Woodland Pond's drivers, stopped by to offer his condolences, even though he knew Anne just slightly.

Thursday, 12 November, the hospital bed and window air conditioner were removed and the bedroom put back the way it was.

Friday, 13 November Jonathan Papin picked up Anne's power chair for Woodland Pond's Rehabilitation Department.

Monday, 16 November at 9AM Dawn Sangrey and Paul Fargis helped me scatter Anne's ashes at the beaver pond.

VSED Narrative

When her ailments overcame her will to live, Anne's sister Joan had died in 2015 at eighty-seven by voluntarily stopping eating and drinking. That may have been the first time we'd heard of or really considered VSED. In 2018, a month shy of his eightieth birthday, a friend and business colleague living in Vermont took advantage of that state's Article 39 Death with Dignity statute, allowing patients with a prognosis of six months or less to live and who qualify to obtain medical aid in dying (MAID). He did and died peacefully without pain in less than an hour.

Despite years of effort, New York still does not have a MAID statute. Even if it did, and even though corticobasal syndrome (CBS) is ultimately fatal, Anne could not get a six month prognosis of death and therefore be eligible to use MAID until long after CBS had robbed her of the physical ability required to self-administer the death causing drug. VSED had been her only option if she wanted to leave life once she could no longer do enough of the things that were important to her.

It's not a happy subject and though we discussed it periodically, those discussions were not in depth. Other than reading Phyllis Shacter's *Choosing to Die*, which made VSED sound simple and painless, our research was superficial. Maybe that was because we didn't want to turn up anything that might suggest there were any potential drawbacks to VSED.

Anne would sometimes ask me, "When should I start to VSED?" My answer was always the same, textbook obvious, "That's up to you. Only you can decide when you can no longer do enough of the things important to you and so want to die." Unstated, but close to the surface, was the strong reaction that thank heavens I don't have to consider that question for myself. I was not nearly as empathetic as I wish I had been

By 2020, many adjustments had been made to make Anne's life easier. Her ability to walk declined and she was largely confined to bed or her power wheelchair. We had gotten a hospital bed which made it possible to raise her back and legs to change position easily to avoid bed sores. She'd also gotten a complex power wheelchair that also had controls to raise the legs and tilt back.

To keep her comfortable and lessen pain, especially at night, we had on hand medical marijuana, Aleve, Tylenol, Ativan, Oxycodone and Quetiapine. But getting Anne settled for bed at night could often take nearly an hour as the bed was adjusted and readjusted; efforts made to get her head comfortable by stuffing rags on either side;

and suitable medications administered. Often, the effort ended, not because we had succeeded, but because our patient was exhausted and just wanted the final bedtime ritual of my reading to her a few pages from C. S. Lewis' *The House at Pooh Corner*. We kissed good night, exchanged "I love yous" and I switched off the light.

When the time came, we were ill-prepared.

At dinner Tuesday evening, 27 October 2020, Anne announced that she would start VSED the next day. I have no recollection of what we had for dinner that night. The next morning, I did have an important early morning doctor's appointment twenty miles away which I knew would take less than an hour. We agreed I should keep that appointment and we notified Hudson Valley Hospice of Anne's plans. Once Anne started to VSED, hospice care would be available to us.

Day One: Wednesday, 28 Oct 20

At midnight, Wednesday evening, Anne took one Ativan and one marijuana. At 1:30AM, she took one Tylenol. Mornings were as they had been for some time. Ana Flores, our primary care giver, arrived each weekday at 7:00AM. Originally from El Salvador, Ana had long dark hair, was short, but very strong with a broad, smiling open face that always invited a smile in response. Her mere presence was always cheering and we both looked forward to her arrivals.

To get Anne up first involved stripping off her urine soaked Assurance which, when tightly folded, fit nicely into a *New York Times* home delivery bag for easy disposal. With warm washcloths, Ana cleaned and dried Anne's perineal area, put on a fresh Assurance, shirt and shorts or slacks and then helped Anne out of bed and into her power chair.

Anne could stand briefly and with Ana's strong support could be turned forty-five degrees and backed into her chair, which I'd brought to the bedroom and up alongside the bed. With a queen sized bed, in which I slept, and the hospital bed next to and parallel with it in our small bedroom, there was little room to maneuver and only about six inches between the chair and the bedroom wall. Nonetheless, Ana managed to get Anne turned, seated and relatively comfortable with her back against the backrest of the chair. With the power chair's controller, I'd then back the chair out from between the bed and wall until it was clear of the bed. This involved care to ensure I did not run over my foot with a chair weighing over three hundred pounds or scrape the wall. Once clear of the bed, the chair could be turned towards the door through which Anne would drive it into the living area.

Ana would make us both a breakfast of granola, all the while maintaining a cheerful banter punctuated with back and forth laughter from all of us. Whatever the weather outside, whatever the private issues she might be having, with us, Ana was always cheerful and upbeat. Before she left at 9:00AM, Ana put the breakfast dishes in the dish-washer, made both beds and folded any towels and cloths that had been used during the night. If need be, she would also put the hamper of dirty clothes in the washer and start that.

This day, I had to leave for my doctor's appointment soon after Ana arrived at 7:00AM. When I returned, Anne was at her computer battling with Dragon's voice recognition software as she dictated emails. The day passed more or less normally with both of us reading or working at our computers. Anne felt neither hunger pangs nor any great urge to drink. She was never a big water drinker, anyway. She didn't even mind watching me eat.

There was inadequate space in either bathroom for Anne to enter in her power chair and then transfer to the toilet. So she used a commode set up in the kitchen when needed. She was still steady enough on her feet so that I alone could help her out of the chair and on and off the commode. Even so, we tried to ensure Anne used the commode when Ana was on hand to help.

Each weekday evening, Ana returned at 5:00PM to organize dinner while we watched a movie. Dinner would be ready by six and made even more appetizing by Ana's care with "presentation." Both Anne and I would sit at the table, but it was no longer as convivial as when Anne was also eating and sharing wine.

After dinner, the major project was getting Anne ready for and into bed. Essentially, this was a reversal of the morning's getting up routine. Turning down the bed; ensuring the waterproof pad was properly positioned on the sheet; undressing Anne; putting on her night gown; and changing her Assurance if needed. Once settled in bed with the back raised just so and perhaps her legs raised slightly as well, the big issue was getting Anne's head comfortable.

At night, she regularly complained of pain at the back of her head. It did not seem to be internal, but we could never quite isolate and eliminate it. We were able to reduce it by using a small inflatable donut to keep the back of her head from pressing on the mattress. Sometimes we tried a heating pad or cold packs, but the donut seemed the most effective. There was also a tendency for Anne's head to loll uncomfortably to the left. So we stuffed old rags and towels on either side of her head to keep it straight. This night, Anne took a single Ativan just before bed.

Day Two: Thursday, 29 Oct 20

At 2:00AM, Anne needed an Ativan tablet, but otherwise seemed to get through the early morning hours okay. In the late morning our hospice nurse and case manager, Sara Tolchin, RN CHPN, visited for the first time. Sara is tall and trim. This we found out only by looking out the window, as she stepped out of her car in our driveway, shivering in the chill while putting on her personal protective equipment (PPE), and then literally rustled up to the door in her paper gown, PPE gown, mask and face shield. As she lamented, the gear required by covid-19 "Puts me at such a remove from my patients. No handshakes; no hugs; and no visible smiles except around the eyes." Anne and I were masked as well, so she couldn't really see us either.

Sara had moved to New York just months before from California, where she had also worked in hospice. But California has had an End of Life Option statute since 2016, leaving Sara with less VSED background. She rose to the occasion and was a hugely empathetic and helpful guide.

Even at our first meeting, Sara sized the situation up accurately. "My first impression of Anne, despite her physical incapacity, is of strength and determination. One of her first questions is, 'How long?' I can see how her disease and the power chair are like a prison to her. She fiercely longs to be set free. And yet, as physically compromised as she is, she is completely in command of the visit. She seems to have no qualms, no misgivings, no shred of uncertainty about her. Some way into our conversation, I learn that it has taken her a year to reach this decision. Now she had decided, she just wanted to *get on with it*. When will it be over?"

We also received from Sara a box, what they called a Comfort Kit, containing various amounts of seven different drugs which could be used for fever, agitation, nausea, vomiting, secretions, anxiety, pain, shortness of breath and constipation. As will be seen, Anne needed only a few of these. But it was nice to have all of them on hand, just in case.

We had been working on the assumption that for Anne to take any water, would be a mistake as it would prolong the process of dying. Sara explained it was important to keep the inside of Anne's mouth moist with, for example, wet sponges on a stick or misting. We found a spray bottle for water used on the orchids which seemed to work much better as we could also spray Anne's face which she often liked and spray directly into her mouth to keep it moist. Once we got this information, we tried to mist the inside of Anne's mouth regularly.

In the afternoon, as arranged by hospice, an oxygen tank and oxygen concentrator were delivered in case of need. When she got back in bed about 6:40PM, Anne took one Ativan, marijuana an hour later and another Ativan at 10:40PM.

Day Three: Friday, 30 Oct 20

Anne had one Ativan at 3:30AM. In the morning, Ana arrived, cheerful as usual. She is our primary, normal link to the outside world and though her news of doings of her extended family – mostly here, but one sister in El Salvador – is usually uneventful, her relatives are at least leading lives not troubled by imminent death.

Anne got up and I had breakfast. At 8:15AM, Kim

Sylvester arrived to shampoo Anne's hair. Kim has the same ebullience and good humor as Ana but is much taller. Hair washing was normally done at the kitchen sink with both Kim and Ana doing a mini ballet around Anne, steadying, washing and drying, all the while the three of them chattering away in a conversation punctuated by many laughs, interruptions and diversions. This may have been one time when Anne could for a few minutes forget that she was busy trying to die.

Even with misting, we had still not figured out the best ways to keep Anne's mouth from becoming too parched. That evening we phoned hospice and the nurse on duty suggested that Anne could rinse her mouth as often as needed with Biotene, for dry mouth. This seemed to help and thereafter, Biotene was kept at Anne's bedside where she could reach it. We also kept a room sized humidifier going in the bedroom to combat the dry air.

At bedtime, Anne took one Ativan tablet followed a few minutes later by a second.

Day Four: Saturday, 31 Oct 20

We had a hard frost overnight, temperature in the twenties with windows glazed with frost and a skim of ice on the bird bath. Anne needed another Ativan at 3:40AM this morning.

As it was Saturday, we would not have Ana, but Gwen Wright came to us at 7AM and stayed until 8PM. We

Skyped with Becca and Ron and Robert and Jill that morning and later in the day, despite the still chill temperature, and because Anne wanted to, we bundled up, put on gloves or mittens, and tooled around the campus in power chairs. It was a tonic for us both to get outside the hospital room atmosphere of our cottage.

Anne took one Ativan at 8PM and another at 11PM.

Day Five: Sunday, 1 Nov 20

Anne had a restless night, taking marijuana by oral syringe at 1:10AM, Ativan tablets at 3 and 3:30AM and more marijuana at 4:30AM. We had no overnight care giver with us this night, so the sleep deprivation wore on both Anne and me. In the morning, her voice was faint.

The day was gray and overcast, but when the temperature got into the high forties, Anne wanted to go out again in the power chairs, even though there was now a light rain. Not to be deterred, we put plastic bags over the chairs' controls and rode out. The trip did not last that long, but at least we got outside briefly which definitely cheered Anne.

In late afternoon, Becca returned from Colorado, having been here from 21 to 26 October. But with Anne in the process of VSED, and despite the great help from care givers, both Anne and I felt Becca's quiet presence and support would both lift our spirits and our ability to cope, which they did. That evening, we watched "The Sound of Music" before dinner.

At 7:55PM, Anne took marijuana followed at 8:12PM by an Ativan tablet; marijuana at 9:35PM; and another Ativan at 9:40PM. With Becca here, we dispensed with the overnight care givers but each time medication was taken, bed clothes and Anne's sleeping position had to be rearranged to get her comfortable. This took some time.

Day Six: Monday, 2 Nov 20

Anne slept fitfully and at 2AM took another Ativan. The day dawned sunny, blustery, windy and cold. Ana arrived at 7AM as usual and was followed this day on Ana's departure at 9AM by the arrival of Kim who was with us for two hours. With Becca's and my help, Kim managed again to wash Anne's hair. Nobody said it but we all sensed it would be the last time.

Sarah came by in mid-afternoon outfitted in her "space suit" and was followed thirty minutes later by Dr. Maggie Carpenter. We were in the kitchen when Anne suddenly said from her powerchair, "I'd really like a gin and tonic." We all laughed and Maggie said, "Tonic would work against VSED. How about just some gin?" to which Anne readily agreed. I poured maybe a half ounce of Tanqueray Rangpur gin into a shot glass which Anne happily downed. We all smiled.

Maggie told us it would now be appropriate for Anne to take one Ativan, 0.25mL morphine and a like amount of marijuana every four hours. If more were needed, doubled doses could be administered every four hours. But when the marijuana ran out, there was no real point in renewing it.

Between 5 and 6PM, Anne had several small sips of iced Tanqueray Rangpur gin

At bedtime at 6:50PM, Anne had Ativan, marijuana and morphine, followed by another Ativan at 9:30PM and then marijuana and morphine at 9:50PM.

Day Seven: Tue, 3 Nov 20

Another fitful night: Ativan at 12:50AM; marijuana and morphine at 2:33AM; and then another Ativan at 3:10AM. That was the last of the marijuana liquid. In addition, Anne rinsed her mouth out with ice water several times during the night. Despite the gin and medications, she and we got little sleep.

By eightish, Anne was up and about in her power chair and perfectly articulate, though a bit confused at times. Her voice was still faint though no fainter than yesterday and when so inclined, she could yell. We thought she might be hanging on for the outcome of the presidential election, although she had never voiced that intent.

On request at 9:15AM, I gave Anne another slug

of gin. Sara came by at 10:15AM and suggested giving medication every four hours rather than just on demand. At 11AM, Anne had two Ativan and an increased dose of 0.5mL of morphine. She had another slug of gin at 12:20PM. This was followed by two Ativan and 0.5mL of morphine at 3PM.

Anne went to bed about 6PM but never got comfortable, even after we had spent considerable time trying to get her head not to loll to the left and to get her spine straighter in the bed. She may have dozed some, but mostly fidgeted, clearly uncomfortable. At 7:20PM and again at 11:07PM Anne had two Ativan and 0.5mL of morphine.

Day Eight: Wed, 4 Nov 20

This was probably the most difficult night for all of us, including Sonia Flores, our overnight care giver, as we were essentially all awake and tending to Anne from 1:18AM until 3:35AM. During this time she variously demanded water, which craving we assuaged with the spray bottle; and wanted to get out of bed and sit in her power chair. We gradually talked her out of that. She had two Ativan and 0.5mL of morphine at 2AM. About 3AM, we gave Anne some water to rinse her mouth. She didn't seem to drink that much, but some. Finally, Anne slept slumped over from 3:30AM until 6:30AM when I got up. Once I was dressed, Becca was up and Anne was awake. Ana arrived at 7:05AM and she and Becca got Anne ready for the day.

The election was still hung up with Biden at 227 and Trump at 213 electoral votes of the 270 needed to declare a winner.

Anne had 1.0mL of morphine at 7:40AM. By 8AM, we had the Brahms "Requiem" conducted by Sir Colin Davis playing in the bedroom. Ana had wiped Anne's mouth, combed her hair and she seemed reasonably comfortable. It was a sunny day with birds flitting about the feeders just outside the windows. Anne made constant demands for water. Ana gave her some sips. I asked her if she wanted to stop VSED. She responded, "No," but continued her demands for water. When I said drinking water would prolong the VSED process, Anne's response was, "Maggie told me I could have all the water I want."

I started sounds of rainfall on an iPhone, hoping that might have a calming effect. Anne was mumbling unintelligibly.

Sara Tolchin came by mid-morning and, in consultation with Maggie Carpenter, prescribed 0.5mL Haldol and 1.0mL morphine every four hours. Anne had her first 0.5mL of Haldol at 10AM, followed at noon by two Ativan and 1.0mL of morphine and this combination had a definite calming effect. At this point, Anne was too weak to swallow liquids or anything else. At 2PM, we administered 0.5mL Haldol under her tongue.

Fortunately, Lorazepam (liquid Ativan) was delivered

at 3:30PM. This now meant that all medications could be delivered via oral syringe under Anne's tongue.

At 4PM, Anne had 0.5mL of Lorazepam and 1.0mL of morphine. About this same time, Becca and I failed to get Anne to and on to the commode fast enough before a bout of diarrhea hit. We cleaned her up as best we could. Fortunately, the more skilled Ana arrived at 5PM and properly cleaned Anne's perineal area, putting on a fresh Assurance and clean nightgown for the night.

For those curious about such matters, a pair of unrinsed and untreated, diarrhea soaked Prana slacks washed alone in a ten year old stock model GE clothes washer came out pristine with the interior of the washing machine spotless as well.

Perhaps it was the introduction of Haldol this morning or it in combination with Lorazepam and the increased morphine dose, but Anne became a lot calmer in the late afternoon.

As a diversion and during all of this, Becca made short order out of putting together an extraordinarily complex wooden jigsaw puzzle, a mere 8.5 by 13 inches but with 254 pieces. The puzzle was of Childe Hassam's painting, "Flags on 57th Street, Winter of 1918." The snow and the multiplicity of flags made it just that much harder.

At 6PM, Anne had another 0.5mL of Haldol followed at 8PM by 0.5mL of Lorazepam and 1.0mL of morphine. We got her much more comfortably situated in bed and she promptly went to sleep.

Day Nine: Thu, 5 Nov 20

At 12:00AM, Anne had 0.5mL Lorazepam and 1.0mL morphine.

At 1:55AM, she awoke and we gave her 0.5mL Lorazepam, 0.5mL Haldol and 1.0mL morphine at 2AM. Minutes later, she coughed and asked, "Can I sit up?" which we accommodated as best we could in Anne's hospital bed. By now, her eyes were closed nearly all the time. But at 2:15AM, they opened and Anne said, "Don't leave me." These were the last words she ever spoke.

By 3AM, Anne was restless but less so than an hour before. Her eyes remained closed all the time now with her mouth gaped open. The inside of her mouth was black which Maggie attributed to dehydration of the membranes in the mouth, despite our efforts to keep the inside of her mouth moist. At 4AM, Anne had 0.5mL Lorazepam and 1.0mL morphine and at 6AM, 0.5mL of Haldol. At 8AM, she had all three drugs in the usual amounts.

Sara visited at 10AM when Anne had another 0.5mL of Haldol. At noon and at 4:00PM she had 0.5mL Lorazepam, 0.5mL Haldol and 1.0mL morphine.

The skin was tightly drawn across Anne's skull and had a waxy yellowish pink tint. She was in or near a coma.

Day Ten: Fri, 6 Nov 20

Anne is clearly in a coma and unresponsive. Becca's and my responsibilities are just to keep her comfortable and administer the same medications under the tongue – 0.5mL Lorazepam, 0.5mL Haldol and 1.0mL morphine at 5:15 and 10:20AM and at 3:30PM, 0.5mL Lorazepam, 1.0mL morphine and 0.5mL Haldol fifteen minutes later.

Sara came by about 10AM and summed up the situation: "At least now that Anne is unresponsive and does not appear to be suffering, I see Ray and Becca relax. No more difficult choices. Now it's just a vigil."

Maggie Carpenter came by around 1PM. We talked quietly, all knowing the end was near.

Sara later wrote, "Day 10 is a Friday and as the workday closes, I have to accept that Anne will die over the weekend when I am off duty and won't be able to do the time of death visit or see her or Ray or Becca again. I concentrate all my energy on wishing her a peaceful passing. I think how much I will miss going there, despite the brevity of our connection and the difficulties of feeling so powerless. I'll miss Ray's morning email, even though it so often detailed a troubled restless night for Anne. I think how the birds will keep on flocking to their feeders outside Anne's windows. Life will go on, despite the gaping hole she leaves."

Day Eleven: Sat, 7 Nov 20

We gave Anne 1.0mL of morphine at 6:40AM and 0.5mL of Lorazepam, 0.5mL of Haldol and 1.0mL of morphine at noon.

About 11:50AM, I learned that Biden had won the election. I immediately told Anne. She gave no response, but I hope she heard me. Later, while Becca and I were having lunch in the kitchen, Becca went to check on Anne. She came back and said simply, "Mom's not breathing." It was about 1:50PM.

We both went back into the bedroom. Anne was not breathing and clearly dead but how could we confirm that? Unskilled taking a pulse, we couldn't even be sure we were taking it in the right place. How could we accurately determine the absence of a pulse? Mirror over the mouth? We didn't get that far.

We phoned hospice, who said the nurse on duty would be over shortly. Gina Law, RN, did arrive soon thereafter. At 2:42PM, she determined officially Anne's death and 2:42PM is the time of death on the Death Certificate.

Gina phoned the funeral home and busied herself dumping all remaining narcotics into a plastic bag partly filled with water, which she took with her on departure.

Not long afterwards, Kim Mangialaschi a slim young lady from the funeral home, arrived in an SUV containing a folding gurney. She backed into our driveway, pulled out the gurney and brought it into the house.

We had already taken off Anne's wedding and amethyst rings and with the help of Gina and me, Kim slid Anne's body into a white body bag and then into a darker bag. We then moved her on to the gurney; Kim wheeled it out; slid it into her SUV; and left.

Aftermath

Loss. Grief. Exhaustion. Emptiness. Relief. Guilt. I'm glad it wasn't me. I could have done more. I could have said this instead of that. I could have been more patient. Why Anne, of all people?

All of that. But omnipresent was a feeling of white hot fury that the only relief an advanced western society could offer a suffering elderly person in Anne's situation was for her to spend an unforeseeable number of days slowly and painfully killing herself by the only means under her control and legally available to her, stopping eating and drinking.

Anne decided to end her life because she could no longer "do" enough of the things important to her and because everything, including the most intimate of daily functions, required help from others. Our society denied her the quick, painless death routinely afforded our pets. Her only legal option was to stop eating and drinking, though the lack of fluid intake is what really caused her death.

Having made and implemented that decision, she was now in a separate world. Nobody was helping her "get better." She was simply being kept as comfortable as possible while awaiting a slow, difficult death. We who loved her could only watch and wait.

Anne had little to do and fewer distractions but to contemplate the process and wonder how long it would take. She was left to concentrate on things like her inability to get comfortable; the itch on her back she couldn't reach; and her thirst. With luck, she would fall asleep for a time and be oblivious. But then she would wake and wonder again how long this is going to take. Her thirst continued, assuaged only slightly by sprays in her mouth. She was maintaining a vigil over her own death.

I had had dogs in my childhood and together, Anne and I had dogs for fifty years; in our children's childhoods, there were also cats and guinea pigs. But dogs were the true members of the family and even though their lives were short, some became more beloved than many humans. But we both knew their times with us were limited and when they could no longer lead enough of the lives that once they led with us and were suffering, we put them down, despite the grief and pain of the loss we felt. We always knew it was the right thing to do.

The worst death was Diggy's, who was only twelve years old when she was diagnosed with lymphoma. She was having increasing trouble breathing, especially at night. Medications provided only slight relief. Finally, both Anne and I knew it was time. But as we drove to the vet's, Diggy exhibited her old vigor and curiosity about her surroundings. Had we made a mistake? Even as we waited in the small room for the vet, Diggy seemed more her old self than like a dog suffering from a pernicious fatal disease. I kept giving her treats as she danced about the room.

The vet arrived and injected a sedative. Diggy skittered around on the polished floor and then finally collapsed on the small mat provided, seemingly totally relaxed. With the next injection, she was gone in minutes. We were desolate and bereft. I gently removed the collar bearing her name and our phone number, put it in my pocket and we left.

Oh, there are some who will go to great lengths to prolong the lives of their pets, whatever the financial costs to them or the uncertain physical and emotional costs to their pets. Within a few miles, we have a cancer treatment center for dogs and cats. We always thought such extreme measures had nothing to do with the welfare of the pets and everything to do with a selfish owner's refusal to let a suffering animal go.

There are safe, painless and quick ways to relieve the suffering of aging and/or ill pets. These are available to humans in some countries and in several states but not all. Nowhere in the United States is medication to end one's life legally available to someone with Anne's disease or those with dementia. It should be.

The days following were filled with the mundane.

Becca set aside those of Anne's clothes and possessions she would like. I reclaimed a treasured and well used thirty or forty year old Patagonia retro jacket Anne had been using because the smooth lining made it much easier for Anne – with help – to get her physically impaired arms in to and out of this jacket.

On Monday morning, 9 November 2020 at 5:15AM, Mike Ennis picked Becca up to drive to the Albany Airport and her return home to Pagosa Springs, CO. Cards and emails of support poured in. I tried in some way to acknowledge them all. One of Woodland Pond's drivers stopped by to offer his condolences. Gifts of food arrived. The hospital bed and like equipment such as a portable room air conditioner were removed and our bedroom rearranged as it was before, now with but a single pillow on our queen sized bed. Anne's power wheelchair was donated to the rehabilitation department at Woodland Pond.

Within a week, I had collected Anne's ashes from the funeral home, where I also got a brief tutorial on crematoria logistics. Despite the Biblical dust to which we are all destined, that's not the product of the crematorium. After cooling, you're left with chunks of bone and possibly pieces of metal – knee or hip replacement parts or pins and screws from bone repairs. These are picked out and the residue ground up so that you do get a lot of dust but also grains or small pebbles of bone. This was put into a thick plastic bag, cinched with a cable tie; and then into a black plastic box. The metric is that one pound of body weight converts to about one square inch of ash.

Anne had wanted her ashes scattered at the beaver pond on Woodland Pond's property. It was there we had first discovered our proximity to beavers, their lodge and where we studied and filmed their activities over several years. We had not been back for some time because the best observation spot was down a steep slope to the shore and this had become increasingly difficult for us to navigate.

I decided that the most accessible place to scatter Anne's ashes would be at the end of the long beaver dam where we had first set up our motion sensitive camera. This was still down a slope, but it was a more negotiable slope.

I enlisted neighbors Dawn Sangrey and Paul Fargis to accompany me as I did not want to risk a solo trip. I had a walking stick and Paul kindly carried the shopping bag containing Anne's ashes, freeing my other hand to grab the support of branches when needed.

The beaver pond is not that big, but to get to the dam side you must go down a wooded slope, cross a trickle of a stream and walk along the pond's edge through thick undergrowth and vines for a hundred yards. I'd forgotten brush clippers which would have been a big help and I nearly tripped on ground roots several times.

At the spot where we'd first put up our motion sensitive camera, Paul handed me the bag of ashes and without ceremony I pitched handfuls into the water. The dust wafted away like an ethereal ghost but the small white pellets of bone disappeared into the pond sand after a mini meteor shower through the clear water at the pond's edge.

Climbing back up the slope I remembered the many times Anne and I had come and gone that way with Anzac and Diggy, especially the return trips. Anzac and Diggy would scamper up and down that slope a dozen times while Anne and I made our laborious climb to the top.

Medical Aid in Dying . . . and More

The first and most important order of business is to achieve the goal of a MAID statute in every state of the union. There is broad national consensus in favor. Achievement just needs legislative will.

Once achieved, proponents can move towards expanding the scope of MAID to include in its scope not just physical health but quality of life factors as well. This will be both a harder sell and more difficult to legislate because there will be few to no objective and quantifiable measures to use.

For the most part, these are not measurable and are solely within the judgment of the individual, such as, independence and the ability to do enough of the things that make one's life worth living. At what point does your dependence upon others for help with basic functions of life become more than you can tolerate? At what point are your physical and/or mental skills so incapacitated that you can no longer do enough of the things that make your life worth living? The individual involved is the only person who can accurately answer those questions.

To broaden MAID, the first rule that would have to be amended would be the requirement for a prognosis of no more than six months until death.

Any expansion of the application of MAID should most heavily impact two forms of disease:

> Those like corticobasal syndrome (CBS) from which my wife suffered. Although neuro-degenerative, these ailments may not significantly impact your mental skills but do affect your physical abilities, gradually stripping muscles of their functionality. For a time, you can devise work-arounds but eventually the cascade of difficulties overcomes you and you want out. You want death while you can still decide and implement (self-administer) your decision as my wife did.

> Those forms of dementia like Alzheimer's and Parkinson's where mental and physical capacity both become compromised. In these cases, you would need to have prepared very specific end of life directives which could be more precisely calibrated as to when they were actionable, using for example the "Functional Assessment Staging Test (FAST)" which defines the stages of Alzheimer's but probably could be applied to other neuro-degenerative diseases.

Your end of life directive could, for example, empower your health care proxy to request euthanasia once you reach level six (affirmed by an appropriate medical professional) on the FAST scale.

To accommodate expansion of MAID to include euthanasia, key points in the common statute might be amended to look like this:

Safeguards:

Only those with an incurable, irreversible and terminal illness confirmed by two doctors are eligible. Individuals are not eligible for medical aid in dying simply because of age or disability.

The attending physician must inform the requesting individual of all their end-of-life options including palliative care, hospice, pain or symptom management and palliative sedation near the end.

A terminally ill individual can withdraw their request for medication, not take the medication once they have it or otherwise change their mind at any point. Similarly, they may decline euthanasia at any point in the process.

If using medical aid in dying rather than requesting euthanasia, the individual must be able to self-administer the medication.

Regulatory and Procedural Requirements:

The individual must make three separate requests for the medication, two oral requests and one written request. Two people must witness the written request, one of whom cannot be a relative or someone who stands to benefit from the person's estate.

If either doctor has concerns about the individual's mental capacity, they must make a referral to a mental health professional for an additional assessment. Medication cannot be prescribed or euthanasia carried out until mental capacity is determined.

Health insurance benefits are unaffected by the availability of medical aid in dying or euthanasia and life insurance payments cannot be denied to the families or beneficiaries of individuals who use the law.

No physician, health provider or pharmacist is required to participate. Those who do participate and comply with all aspects of the law are given civil and criminal immunity.

Anyone attempting to coerce an individual will face criminal prosecution.

Unused medication must be disposed of according to the guidelines specified by the U. S. Food and Drug Administration.

The state Department of Health is required to

issue a publicly available annual report. Identifying information about individual patients and doctors is kept confidential.

The underlying illness – not medical aid in dying or euthanasia – will be listed as the cause of death on the Death Certificate.

Medications Dispensed

Book MAID/Meds Dispensed One										
Medications Dispensed										
VSED Day										
Day	Thu		Fri	Sat		Sun			Mon	
Date (2020)	22-Oct		23-Oct	24-Oct		25-Oct			26-Oct	
Time [Hrs|Mins]	10:15	20:30	20:30	20:30	21:05	1:00	10:00	20:00	2:00	19:50
Aleve 220mg tabs	2									
Ativan 5mg tabs						1				
Lorazepam										
Gin										
Haldol										
Marijuana		1	1	1				1	1	1
Morphine										
Oxycodone 5mg tabs					1					
Quetiapine 25mg tabs							1			
Tylenol 500mg tabs				1						

VSED Day			2			1			
Day			Thu			Wed			Tue
Date (2020)			29-Oct			28-Oct			27-Oct
Time [Hrs:Mins]	22:40	19:50	18:40	02:00	18:30	1:30	0:00	19:05	2:00	0:00
Aleve 220mg tabs										
Ativan 5mg tabs	1		1	1	1		1	1		
Lorazepam										
Gin										
Haldol										
Marijuana		1					1			1
Morphine										
Oxycodone 5mg tabs										
Quetiapine 25mg tabs										
Tylenol 500mg tabs						1			2	

VSED Day	3	3	3	4	4	4	5	5	5	5
Day	Fri	Fri	Fri	Sat	Sat	Sat	Sun	Sun	Sun	Sun
Date (2020)	30-Oct	30-Oct	30-Oct	31-Oct	31-Oct	31-Oct	1-Nov	1-Nov	1-Nov	1-Nov
Time [Hrs:Mins]	3:30	18:55	19:01	3:41	20:00	23:00	1:10	3:00	3:30	4:30
Aleve 220mg tabs										
Ativan 5mg tabs	1	1	1	1	1	1		1	1	
Lorazepam										
Gin										
Haldol										
Marijuana							1			1
Morphine										
Oxycodone 5mg tabs										
Quetiapine 25mg tabs										
Tylenol 500mg tabs										

VSED Day	5				6				7	
Day		Sun			Mon				Tue	
Date (2020)		1-Nov			2-Nov				3-Nov	
Time [Hrs:Mins]	19:55	20:12	21:35	21:40	2:00	18:50	21:30	21:50	0:50	2:33
Aleve 220mg tabs										
Ativan 5mg tabs		1		1	1	1	1		1	
Lorazepam										
Gin					16:30gin					
Haldol										
Marijuana	1		1			1		1		1
Morphine						0.25mL		0.25mL		0.25mL
Oxycodone 5mg tabs										
Quetiapine 25mg tabs										
Tylenol 500mg tabs										

VSED Day	7							8		
Day								Wed		
Date (2020)								4-Nov		
Time [Hrs:Mins]	3:10	9:15	11:00	12:20	15:00	19:20	23:07	2:00	7:40	10:00
Aleve 220mg tabs										
Ativan 5mg tabs (1)			2		2	2	2	2		
Lorazepam										
Gin		gin		gin						
Haldol										0.5mL
Marijuana										
Morphine			0.5mL		0.5mL	0.5mL	0.5mL	0.5mL	1.0mL	
Oxycodone 5mg tabs										
Quetiapine 25mg tabs										
Tylenol 500mg tabs										

	12:00	14:00	16:00	18:00	20:00	0:00	2:00	4:00	6:00	8:00
VSED Day	8					9				
Day	Wed					Thu				
Date (2020)	4-Nov					5-Nov				
Time [Hrs:Mins]	12:00	14:00	16:00	18:00	20:00	0:00	2:00	4:00	6:00	8:00
Aleve 220mg tabs										
2 Ativan 5mg tabs										
Lorazepam			0.5mL		0.5mL	0.5mL	0.5mL	0.5mL		0.5mL
Gin										
Haldol		0.5mL		0.5mL			0.5mL		0.5mL	
Marijuana										
Morphine	1.0mL		1.0mL		1.0mL	1.0mL	1.0mL	1.0mL		1.0mL
Oxycodone 5mg tabs										
Quetiapine 25mg tabs										
Tylenol 500mg tabs										

	VSED Day 9									Totals
Day	Thu	Thu	Thu	Fri	Fri	Fri	Sat	Sat	Sat	
Date (2020)	5-Nov	5-Nov	5-Nov	6-Nov	6-Nov	6-Nov	7-Nov	7-Nov	7-Nov	
Time [Hrs:Mins]	10:00	12:00	16:00	5:15	10:20	15:30	15:45	6:40	12:00	
Aleve 220mg tabs										440mg
Ativan 5mg tabs										170mg
Lorazepam			0.5mL	0.5mL	0.5mL		0.5mL			6mL
Gin										
Haldol	0.5mL		0.5mL	0.5mL	0.5mL		0.5mL		0.5mL	6.5mL
Marijuana										14 caps
Morphine			1.0mL	1.0mL	1.0mL	1.0mL		1.0mL	1.0mL	18.25mL
Oxycodone 5mg tabs										5mg
Quetiapine 25mg tabs										0mg
Tylenol 500mg tabs										2,000mg

The Process of Dying

In my youth, death of elderly relatives was always distant. My immediate family lived in New York state and nearly all close relatives lived in the South. My grandparents died but I was spared details.

My first close family encounter with death occurred during the summer I graduated from college. A massive heart attack killed my father at work. He was fifty-four years old. He did have a weakened heart, but there was no steady decline beforehand and none of us were at the scene when it occurred.

Twenty-five years later, my mother may have had a stroke, tumbled down a flight of stairs and was in a coma. She was in the ICU hooked up to a ventilator and other machines that kept her vital functions working. Finally, doctors assured us she would not recover and, after a family conference, we disconnected the machines and she died peacefully.

Rarely does death of the elderly occur so "cleanly" or expeditiously. Usually, it's preceded by slow deterioration, which may be accelerated by one or more of the ailments that can eventually overtake so many of us – heart problems, blood pressure, obesity, diabetes, cancer, pneumonia, joint replacements, hearing and eyesight issues, Alzheimer's, Parkinson's and other neuro-degenerative diseases.

Even if you escape all those accelerants, you will still face the slow, steady decline of just getting older.

For me, it became noticeable about age eighty. I'd been a runner for many years and that had adversely impacted my knees. One was replaced; the other should be. Recovering from my knee replacement was my first experience with a wheeled walker. We did short hikes with our dogs and usually once a week we met friends for a three hour hike and geocaching expedition followed by lunch. Gradually, these hikes got harder; my stamina wasn't what it once was. Increasingly, I had to sit down frequently. After a few more years, I could only hike for about an hour at one go. The lunches I could still easily do.

At ages seventy-eight, Anne and I had signed up for a cottage at Woodland Pond at New Paltz (NY), a continuing care retirement community (CCRC). We got very involved in activities there, even though we remained in our home eight miles away. We also saw more and more of "the future."

These don't normally appear in the publicity for retirement communities but we saw fellow residents using canes, walking sticks, walkers and wheelchairs, some battery powered. Most of our fellow residents looked well north of sixty-five rather than the beautifully coiffed and attractive folks pictured in the brochures who looked annoyingly more like forty-five . . . and ready for an afternoon of singles tennis or touch football.

Muscular strength declines and arthritis which few of us escape takes a major toll on finger dexterity. Having once had only a primary care physician, you gradually find yourself involved with multiple specialists – cardiology, neurology, dermatology, ophthalmology, urology, audiology, etc. You need more sleep and may even start taking afternoon naps to be alert for evening activities (which, even so, often end by 9PM).

Independence and the ability to live independently become more important, whether in your own home or in the congregate setting of a CCRC. To that end, concerns about balance become an increasing issue. You do exercises or take classes to improve balance. The great fear is that a fall could easily break an arm, leg or hip and destine you to weeks of rehabilitation or, worse, be the beginning of a more rapid decline.

Even though we have on site assisted living, skilled nursing, memory care units and a rehabilitation center, nobody wants to go there (except maybe to rehab) if they can possibly avoid it.

Standing or walking longer distances becomes painful. You need to sit more or at least know just where the nearest chair is. Then there are varying grades of incontinence.

You must manage sudden, uncontrollable urges to urinate. This is not likely to get better or easier. For some degree of confidence, you may resort to wearing Depends or Assurance to avoid the public embarrassment of peeing your pants.

Endemic memory issues are difficult and annoying. You stand to get something from the next room but by the time you get there, you can't remember what you were going for. Your speech may slow or you can't quickly find the right word when speaking.

Modern medicine can patch up many of these issues. But you may notice your doctors now talk less of "cure" or "back to your old self" and more about "stabilizing" or "slowing" something. As an example, my ophthalmologist now speaks only of trying to ensure that my eyes "last longer than I do."

There are also non-medical aids available to the aging to help keep them in the game. If arthritis or some other affliction make it difficult to hold books or turn pages, audio books proliferate. Similarly, if your fingers are no longer as adept on a keyboard, voice recognition software makes dictating emails, memos or texts increasingly accurate and fast.

For the most part, we live longer and more and more issues of the elderly can be alleviated. But there may come a point where the combination of ailments, declining abilities, etc. may make your life no longer worth living. The tipping point might be when your dependence on others to take care of too many of your basic needs simply becomes more than you can tolerate, making your life no longer worth living.

Even if your state has a MAID statute, you wouldn't qualify unless you had a prognosis of six months or less to live.

Your only option would be to voluntarily stop eating and drinking (VSED). But that's drawn out, uncomfortable, painful and grossly unpleasant to you and your loved ones.

Could not the terms of MAID be expanded to consider "quality of life?" Of necessity, that would have to be subject to each individual's interpretation as to when their quality of life had declined to the extent that life was no longer worth living. Otherwise, it would also/could also incorporate the same safeguards and restrictions – absent the six month prognosis of death – that surround existing MAID statutes.

Failure to expand MAID coverage does not make the underlying issues go away. It just forces the patient back on to VSED and may also force them to use it sooner than they might prefer, simply to do so before they have lost the mental ability to follow through.

Bills to expand MAID coverage along these lines had been introduced in California (2015) and more recently in Oregon. Neither got much traction and opposition was strong. But as baby boomers age we may become more comfortable with what other countries have done and are doing regarding both medical aid in dying and euthanasia.

The difference between the two has largely to do with who administers the final, fatal dose that brings about death. MAID requires that the individual self-administer the dosage, in part to ensure that it is being ingested entirely voluntarily. The process is only facilitated by a doctor who prescribes the necessary medicines.

With euthanasia, the fatal dose is administered by someone other than the suffering individual, often by a doctor. If euthanasia is performed at the request of the patient it can be termed "voluntary euthanasia."

Euthanasia and medical aid in dying are legal in the Netherlands, Belgium, Luxembourg, Canada and Colombia. As recently as 2021, Portugal's parliament voted overwhelmingly to legalize euthanasia under strict rules.

At the other extreme is the United Kingdom, where euthanasia can lead to a charge of murder and medical aid in dying a sentence of up to fourteen years in prison for the aider. Anonymous surveys suggest that euthanasia does occur in the UK but that it is relatively rare.

Nonetheless, the UK provides us with a particularly sensational example that remained a secret for fifty years. A page one article by Joseph Lelyveld in *The New York Times* of 28 November 1986 carried the lead: "As he lay comatose on his deathbed in 1936, King George V was injected with fatal doses of morphine and cocaine to assure him a painless death in time, according to his physician's [Lord Dawson's] notes, for the announcement to be carried in the morning papers rather than the less appropriate evening journals." Of further significance, also according to Lord Dawson's notes, was the fact that the King's wife, Queen Mary, and his son, who would succeed him as Edward VIII, told the doctor "they did not want the King's life needlessly prolonged if his illness was clearly fatal."

Other Resources

Blackbird, a film directed by Roger Michell starring Susan Sarandon and Kate Winslet, 2019.

Chabot, Boudewijn, *Dignified Dying: A Guide, Death at Your Bidding*, Zutphen, Netherlands: CPI/Kroninklijke Wöhrmann, 2015.

Chabot, Boudewijn, *Stopping Eating and Drinking: A Guide*, Amsterdam, Netherlands: Foundation Dignified Dying, 2014.

Compassion & Choices, 101 SW Madison St Ste 8009, Portland, OR 97207, 800 247-7421, compassionand-choices.org

Coombs Lee, Barbara, *Finish Strong: Putting Your Priorities First at Life's End*, Littleton, CO: Compassion & Choices, 2019.

deMaine, Jim, *Facing Death: Finding Dignity, Hope and Healing at the End*, Bellevue, WA: Clyde Hill Publishing, 2020.

End Game, a documentary directed by Rob Epstein and Jeffrey Friedman, 2018.

End of Life Choices New York, 244 Fifth Ave Ste 2010, New York, NY 10001, 212 726-2010, info@endofli-fechoicesny.org, endoflifechoicesny.org

Englehart, Katie, *The Inevitable: Dispatches on the Right to Die*, New York, NY: St. Martin's Press, 2021.

Humphry, Derek, *Final Exit: The Practicalities of Self-Deliverance and Assisted Suicide for the Dying*, New York, NY: Delta Trade Paperbacks, 2019.

Loisel, Laurie, *On Their Own Terms: How One Woman's Choice to Die Helped Me Understand My Father's Suicide*, Amherst, MA: Levellers Press, 2019.

Miller, BJ and Berger, Shoshana, *A Beginner's Guide to the End: Practical Advice for Living Life and Facing Death*, New York, NY: Simon & Schuster, 2019.

Nitschke, Philip and Stewart, Fiona, *The Peaceful Pill Handbook*, Blaine, WA: Exit International USA, 2019.

Shacter, Phyllis, *Choosing to Die: A Personal Story, Elective Death by Voluntarily Stopping Eating and Drinking (VSED) in the Face of Degenerative Disease*, Middletown, DE: CreateSpace, 2017.

Shavelson, Lonny, *A Chosen Death: The Dying Confront Assisted Suicide*, New York, NY: Simon & Schuster, 1995.

Acknowledgments

Of inestimable value was the unconditional support both Anne and I received from our two children and their partners, Randy Smith, Wanda Beaudry Kelly, Becca Smith and Ron Decker.

Anne's care givers, Ana Flores, Kim Sylvester, Gwen Wright and Sonia Flores sustained both of us with their laughter, good humor, empathy and skills when we were in extremis. We could not have coped without them.

When Anne started VSED, Hudson Valley Hospice mobilized on our behalf. We were also fortunate that their medical director for Ulster County, Dr. Maggie Carpenter, had been Anne's primary care physician for the previous two years. Our case manager was Sara Tolchin, RN CHPN, who could not have been more caring or attentive to Anne's needs and concerns. They were backed by an effective support staff.

Carol O'Biso, Larry and Marla Randall provided crucial help with the front cover's design and photography and Gretchen Daum took the back cover photo.

Friends and relatives around the globe were a continuing boost on dark days, especially the staff and residents of Woodland Pond at New Paltz (NY), the continuing care retirement community where we live. That concern and support of me continues to this day.

About the Author

Ray Smith graduated from Washington and Lee University with a B.A. in English, *magna cum laude* and Phi Beta Kappa. This was followed by a year in France as a Fulbright Scholar; a tour with the Army in Germany; and a long career as a commercial banker, in New York City and London.

He and Anne raised two children during a marriage that spanned sixty years.

CPSIA information can be obtained
at www.ICGtesting.com
Printed in the USA
FSHW010046240421

9 781954 744134